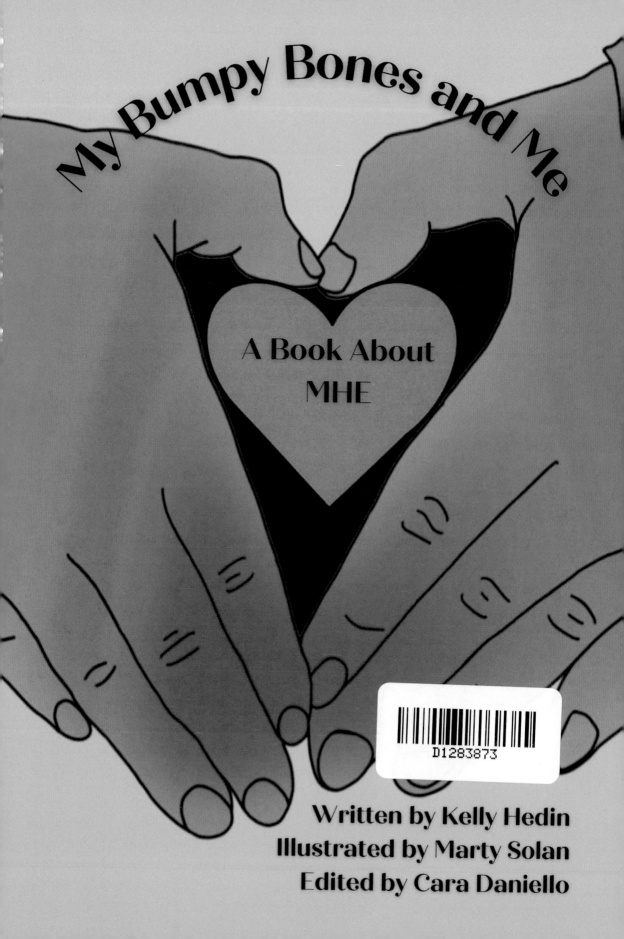

My Bumpy Bones and Me

A Book About MHE

Written by Kelly Hedin
Illustrated by Marty Solan
Edited by Cara Daniello

ISBN: 978-0-578-38532-7

Front cover image by Marty Solan.
Illustrations by Marty Solan.
Book design by Cara Daniello.

Printed by Amazon, in the United States of America.

First printing edition 2022.

hedink3@gmail.com

I dedicate this book to my loving family – my inspiration, my muses, my everythings. With your love and support, you have made my dream of becoming an author a reality.
- K. H.

Hi! My name is Riley, and this is my sister Reese. We have MHE. "What is MHE?" you ask. Well, MHE stands for Multiple Hereditary Exostoses, and it's a rare bone disease. MHE causes benign tumors to grow on your bones. The fun term that we like to call it is "bumpy bones."

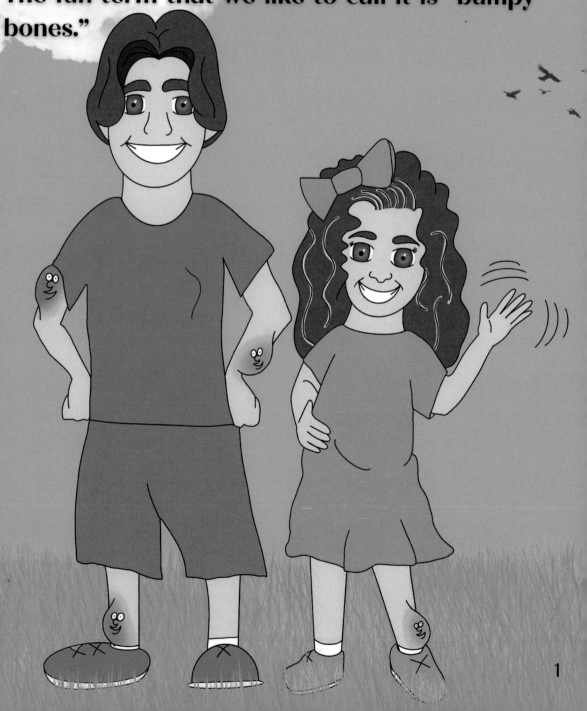

Doctor's Office

My sister and I found out we have MHE when we were each three years old. Our mom took us to the doctor because she saw a bump on our ribs.

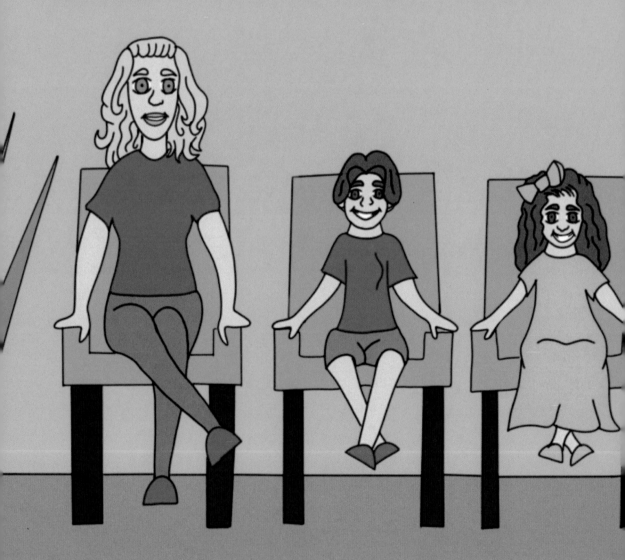

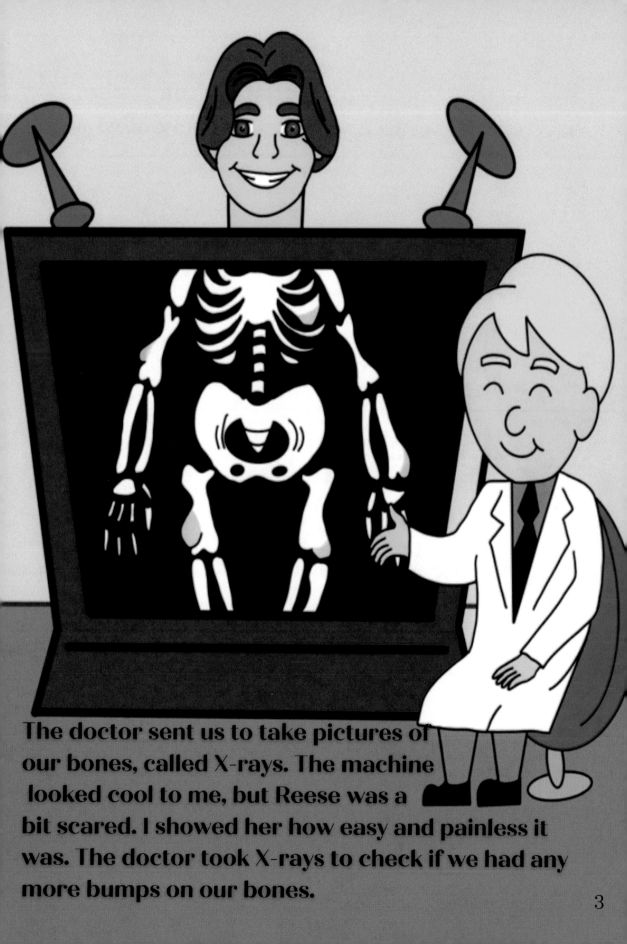

The doctor sent us to take pictures of
our bones, called X-rays. The machine
looked cool to me, but Reese was a
bit scared. I showed her how easy and painless it
was. The doctor took X-rays to check if we had any
more bumps on our bones.

3

The doctors told my mom that the tumors we have on our bones are called osteochondromas.

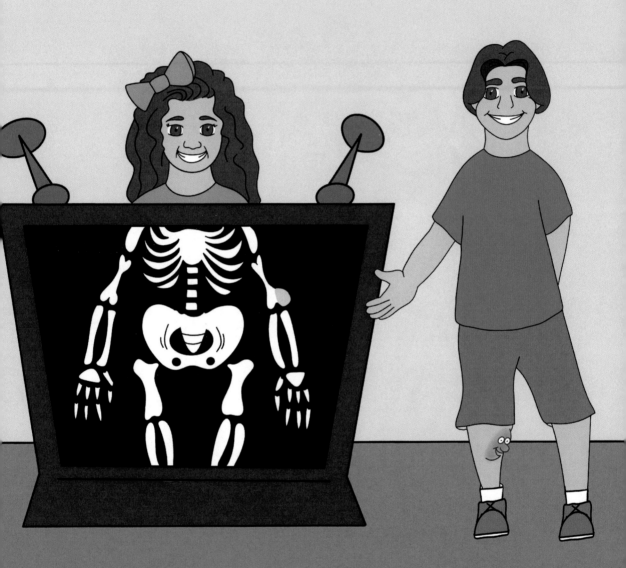

They can make your bones look different. Sometimes your bones don't match and they can be different sizes.

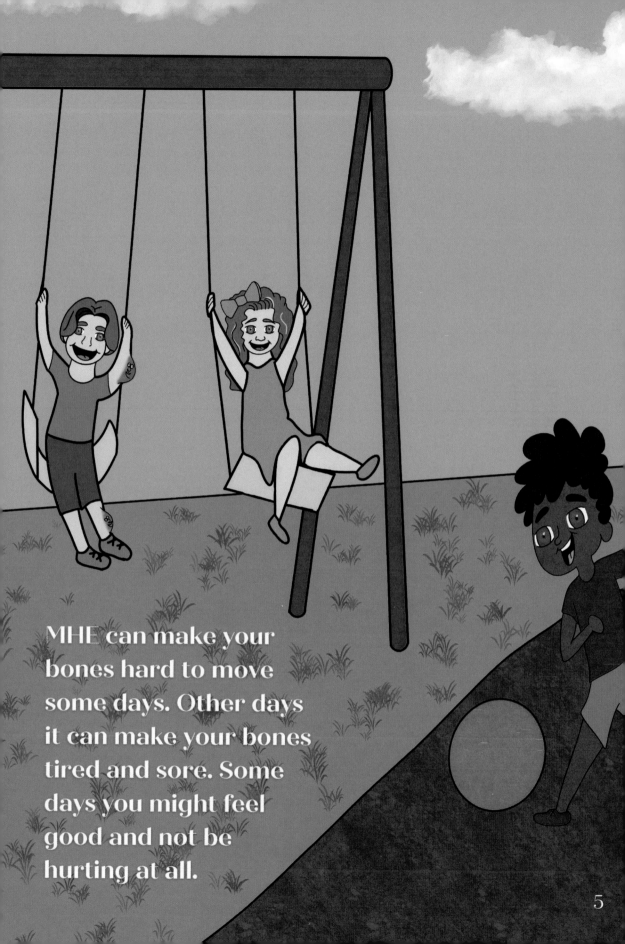

MHE can make your bones hard to move some days. Other days it can make your bones tired and sore. Some days you might feel good and not be hurting at all.

We learned that the MHE tumors grow differently in everyone.

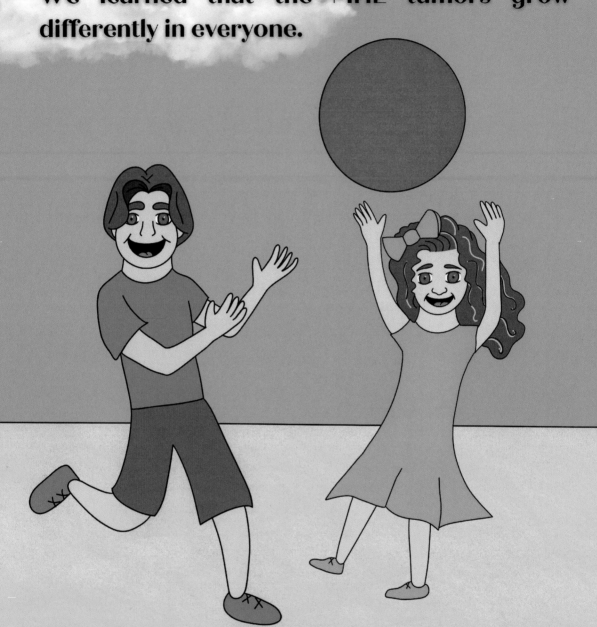

I have over 100 tumors in my body, and Reese has about 10. The tumors grow mostly on your longer bones, like your arm and leg bones.

The tumors can be small or big, and you can see the bumps (that's why we call them bumpy bones). Some can grow on the inside of your bones and you can only see them in the special pictures like X-rays.

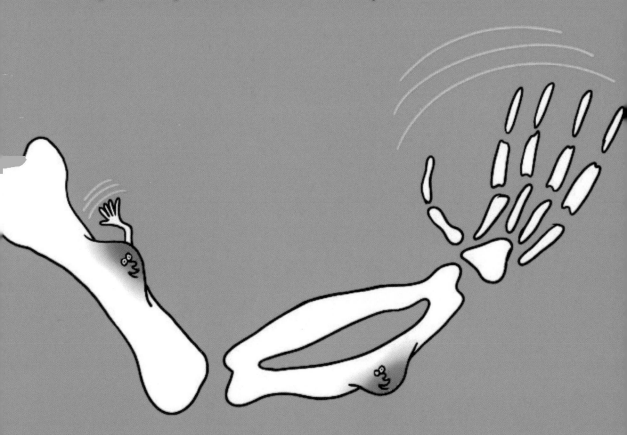

MHE is a rare bone disease, affecting 1 out of every 50,000 people at birth. As I said before, Reese and I got diagnosed with MHE at the age of three. I'm 12 now, and Reese is 9. With MHE being so rare, my mom says this makes us some pretty special kids.

MHE is mostly hereditary, which means that it gets passed down in your family, like certain eye or hair colors.

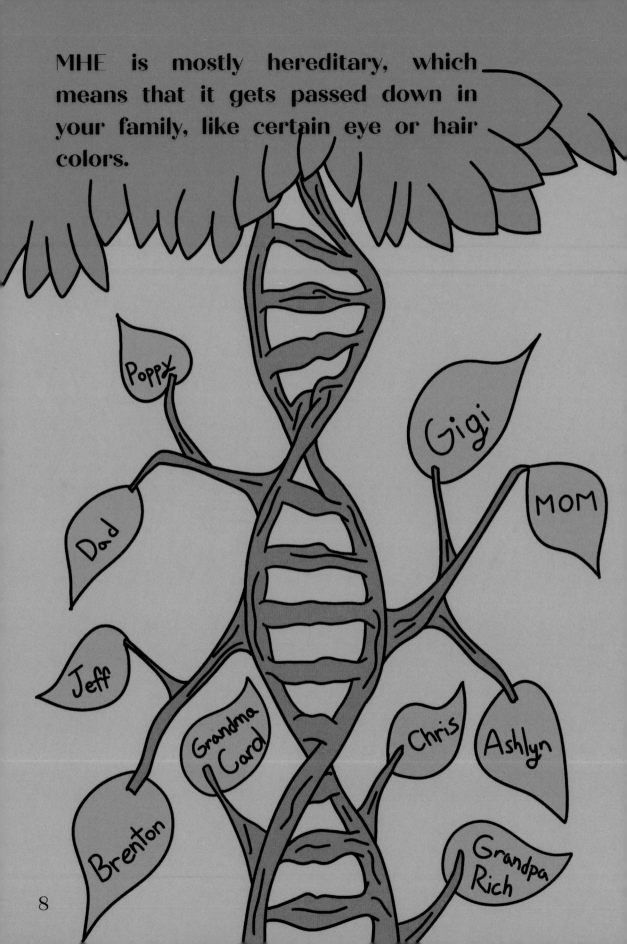

The doctors call the type that isn't hereditary "spontaneous MHE," which means that some people get it without the disease running in their families. Only 10% of all people who have MHE have the spontaneous type.

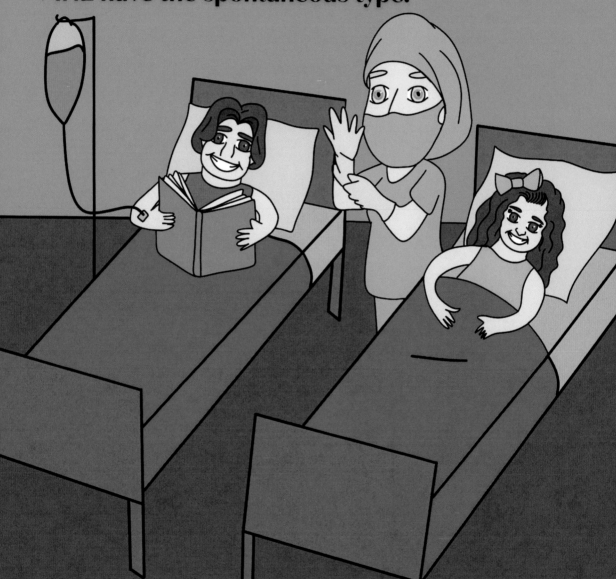

Reese and I have both had some surgeries to make us feel better and help our bones move more easily.

Sometimes my friends ask me questions about MHE. One day my friend Garrett asked me, "Why do your bones stick out like that?" It might make some people feel weird to be asked about their bumpy bones, but I knew Garrett just wanted to make sure that I was okay.

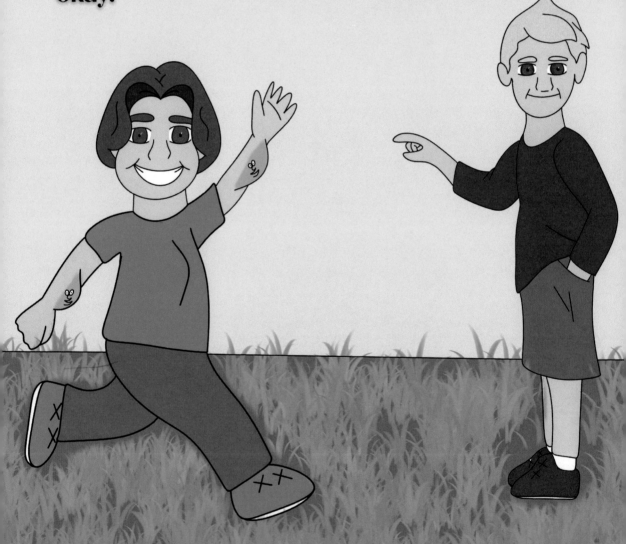

I told Garrett it's because I was born this way, so I have bumpy bones. They just grow differently than other people's bones.

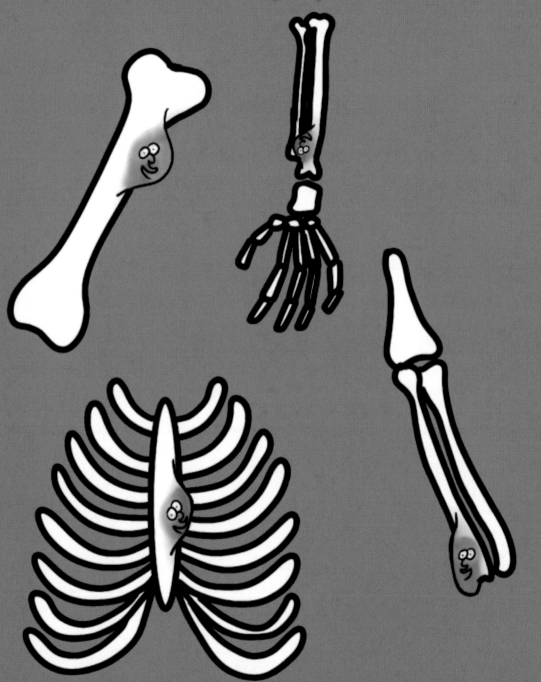

Sometimes I even give them funny names so they're less scary.

Then Garrett asked me if my bumpy bones hurt. I said, "Sometimes they do. It depends on where the bumps are. Other times they just look more painful than they really are."

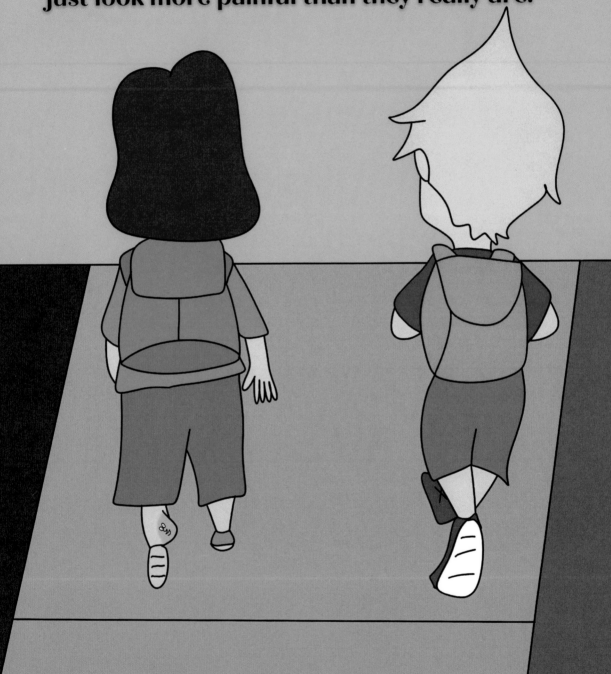

I told Garrett I can do all the same things he can, but sometimes my bones get tired and hurt, so I just stop and rest.

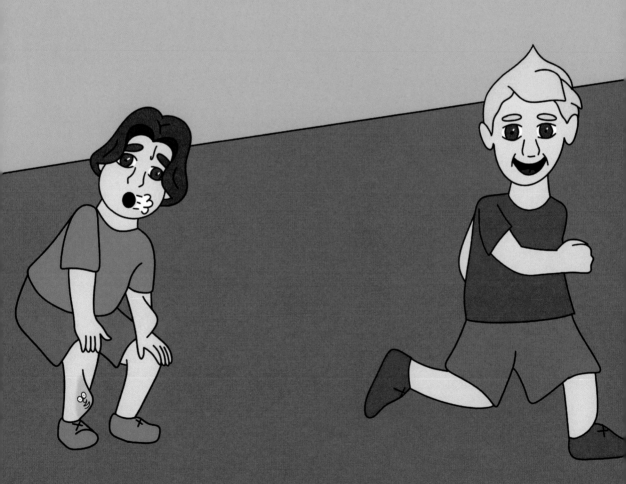

Garrett asked me about a cure for MHE or if the bumps could go away on their own. I repeated what I learned from the doctor. "No," I said, "they don't go away, unless you have surgery."

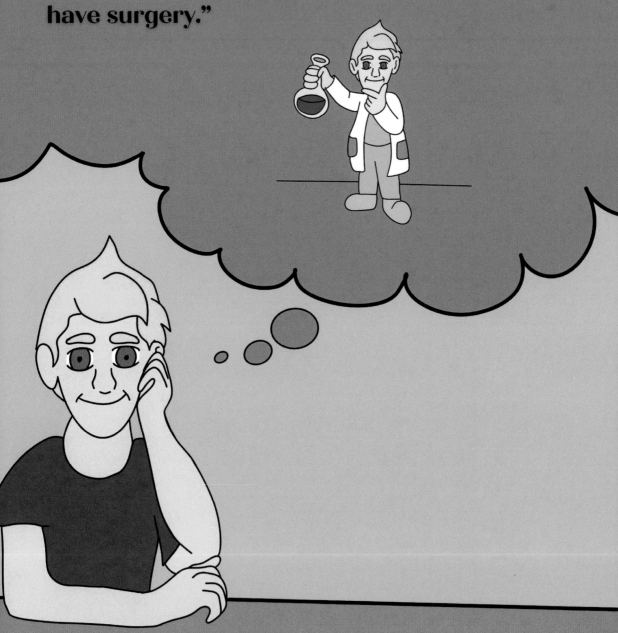

"Surgery?" Garrett gasped. "That sounds scary."

"No," I explained, "there are a lot of people in the hospital that help you and tell you everything so they make sure it's not scary at all. Plus they let your parents stay with you. And you can even get ice cream when it's done!"

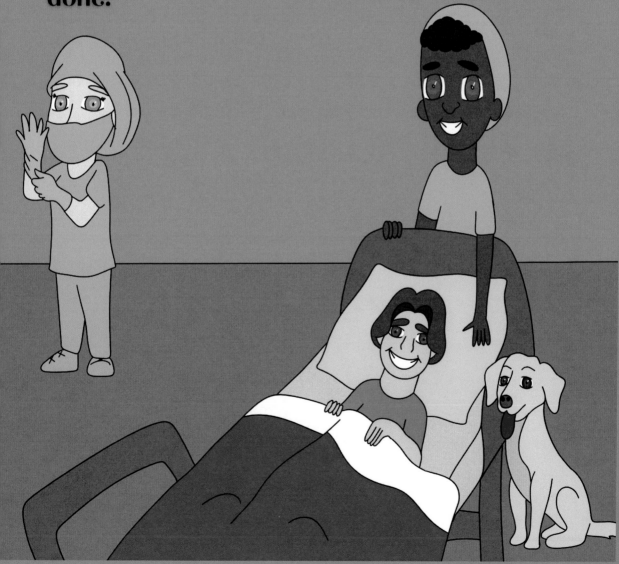

I've had five surgeries already, and Reese has had one. When we go to the hospital, we get our own room. The doctor comes in and tells us which bumps they're going to take out.

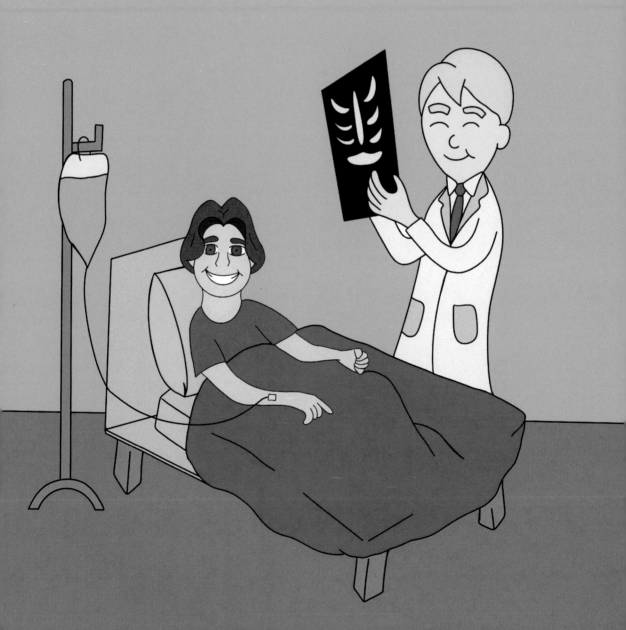

"What happens next?" Garrett asked.

"Well, they take our temperature and make sure our heart rate is good. They even put a cool monitor on your finger to keep track of it. It makes me feel like a robot!"

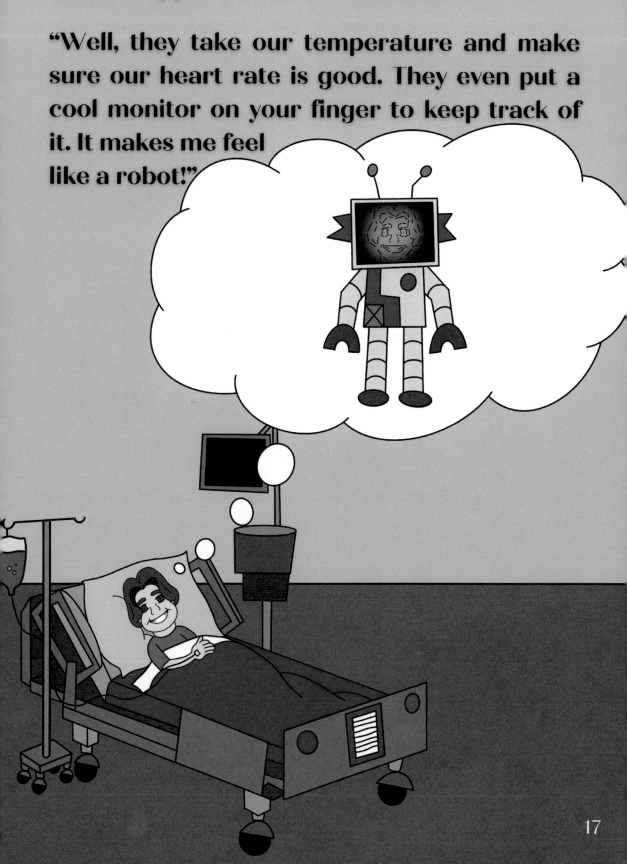

"Does it hurt?" Garrett wanted to know.

"Nope, not at all. You sleep the whole time when the doctor takes the bumps out. Before they take you into the surgery room, they give you what my mom calls 'giggle juice' to make sure you stay asleep, and it helps you not to worry."

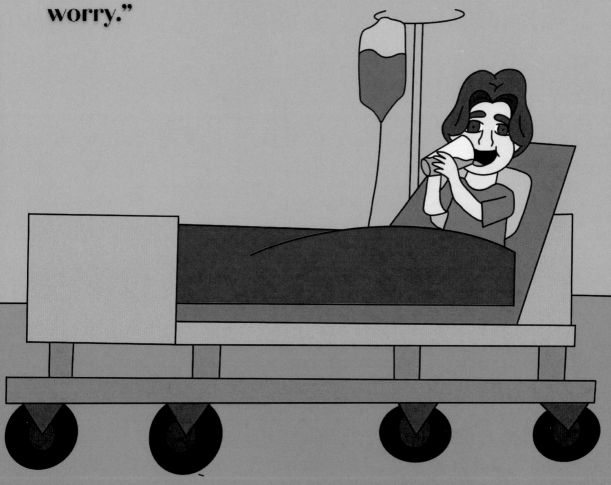

During my last surgery, I had an external fixator put into bone to make it grow.

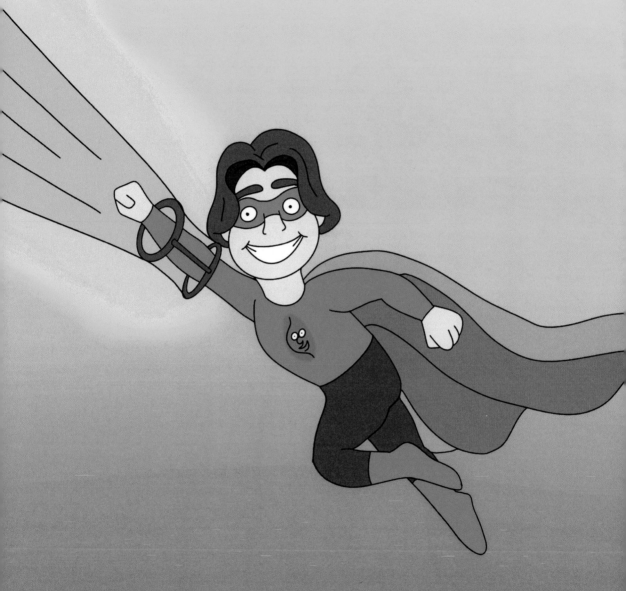

It looked pretty cool, and it make me feel like a superhero!

Reese had surgery on her elbow and arm. She has an internal fixator to help her bone grow. She wore a cast for 8 weeks when she was done, and she had all of our friends and family sign it.

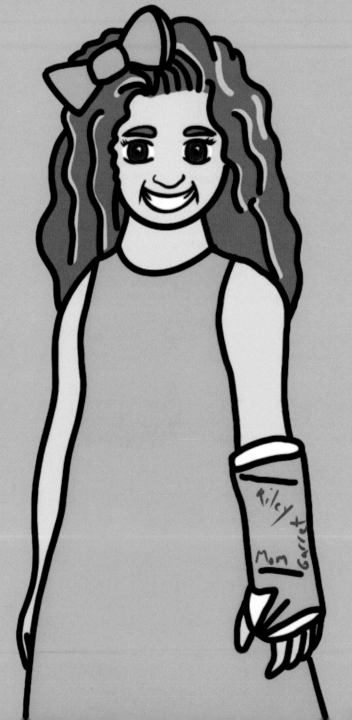

Anyway, MHE is different in everyone, even for Reese and me.

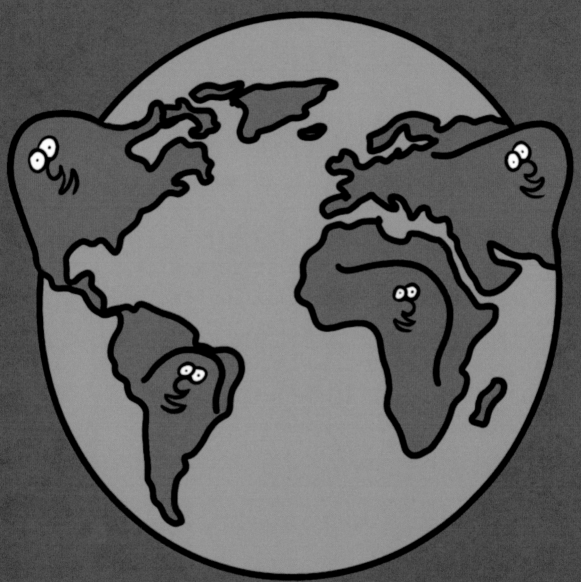

It's something that hopefully in the future there will be a cure for. MHE is diagnosed all over the world, and my mom, Reese, and I are working hard to help more people understand what it is.

Living with MHE can be tough, but overall you can live a healthy, active, and fulfilled life. Bumpy bones and all.

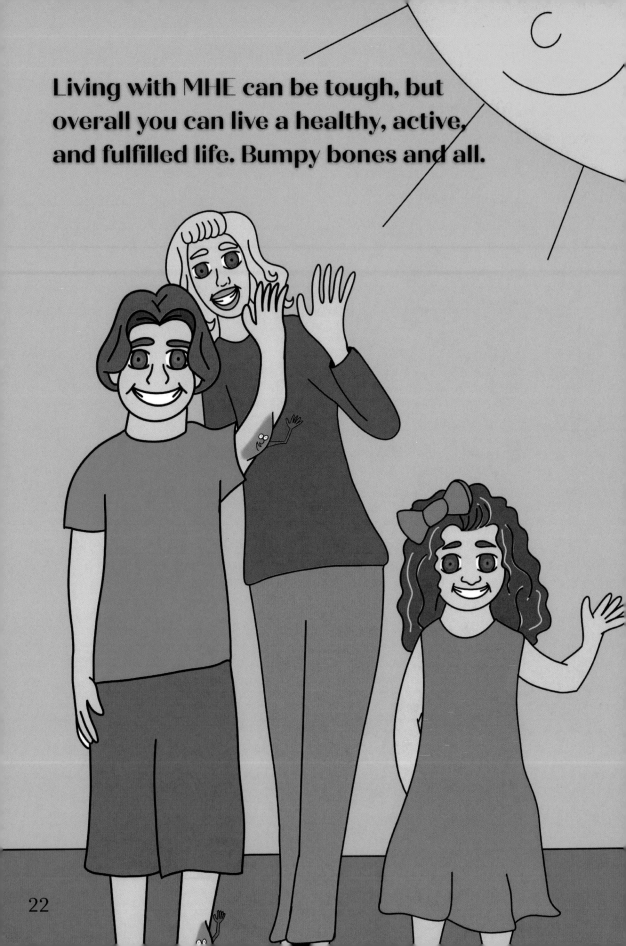

About the Author

Kelly Hedin is thrilled to be breaking into children's literature with her debut book, *My Bumpy Bones and Me*. Kelly lives in Toms River, New Jersey, with her loving husband Jeff, and together they are raising 5 amazing children. Kelly teaches high school physical education and health and has changed the lives of countless students over the past 20 years. *My Bumpy Bones and Me* is inspired by two of her children who have MHE. Kelly hopes this book helps children and their families become more familiar with and better educated about MHE. This book is the resource she wishes she had when her children were first diagnosed and is grateful to pass along her knowledge to families sharing similar experiences as hers. Stay strong, bumpy bones and all!

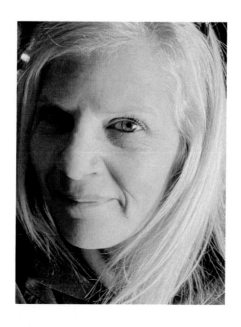